Alone for 40 Days

A Step-by-Step Guide to Physical, Mental, and Spiritual Renewal Through Solitude Without Feeling Lonely

Dr. MT Raza

Dr. MT Raza

Alone for 40 Days

A Step-by-Step Guide to Physical, Mental, and Spiritual Renewal Through Solitude Without Feeling Lonely

PUBLISHED BY: Dr MT Raza

Introduction of the Book: Alone for 40 days

Welcome, readers, to <u>Alone for 40 Days</u>, a guide crafted to lead you on a journey toward holistic renewal. This book takes you through the powerful experience of solitude as a means of reconnecting with yourself and nourishing your mind, body, and spirit. Spending time alone, as outlined in this guide, is not about isolation but about creating space to discover, reflect, and recharge without the weight of loneliness. Through each chapter, you'll find structured exercises, reflective prompts, and actionable insights to help you build a balanced approach to self-renewal.

To make your journey even more effective, I've developed two accompanying resources—a **Planner**, <u>the 40-Day Solitude Planner</u> (Available at amazon KDP) and **a Notion Template**, <u>40 Days of Clarity</u> (available at gumroad.com), that expand on the exercises and principles in this book. These tools are designed to bring added structure and motivation to your 40-day experience. The Weekly Planner, available as a convenient KDP printable, will be your go-to for setting daily intentions, tracking your progress, and jotting down reflections. You'll find spaces for goal setting, habit tracking, and guided journaling, making it an ideal complement to your solitude journey. The Notion Template, on the other hand, offers a digital approach for those who prefer organizing and recording their experiences online. Complete with habit trackers, mood logs, and integrated reflections, this template allows you to keep everything in one place, accessible from anywhere.

To enhance your journey through this book, we've included a **mind map** at the end of the book, that visually organizes the core concepts, stages, and strategies presented in *Alone for 40 Days*. This mind map is designed to serve as a quick-reference guide, offering several benefits: retention and recall, big picture understanding, engagement and clarity

In addition to these resources, I'd like to invite you to join the Alone for 40 Days **Telegram community**: <u>Alone for 40 Days</u>. Here, you'll find a supportive network of like-minded individuals who are also on their own journeys toward personal renewal. This is a space for sharing progress, exchanging insights, and asking questions as we go through the 40 days together. Whether you're looking for encouragement, feedback, or simply a place to reflect on your experiences with others, this channel offers a positive environment for building connections and enhancing your understanding of solitude.

Finally, I invite you to join our community on Telegram: Alone for 40 Days. Here, you'll find a supportive space to share your journey with others who are on a similar path. Engage in discussions, share progress, and exchange insights as we navigate this 40-day journey together. Whether you're diving into the book, using this planner, or exploring the Notion template, this channel will serve as a valuable resource for connection and inspiration.

Personalized Notion Template Offer: In addition to the Weekly Planner and Notion Template, I'm excited to offer a personalized service for readers interested in further tailoring their habit-building experience. If you'd like a customized Notion template built around your unique goals and routines, simply reach out through the Telegram channel. Together, we'll create a toolkit designed specifically for you, offering the most practical support in tracking and reinforcing the habits you wish to build.

This journey is about more than 40 days—it's about creating a life filled with intention, resilience, and joy. May these tools and resources serve you well on your path.

Sections Symbols

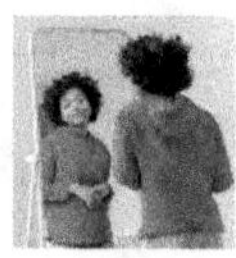

Reflect Prompt

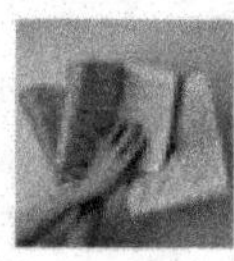

Personal Story

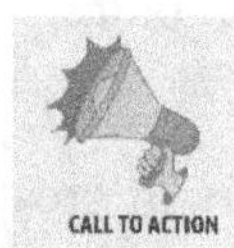

Call to Action

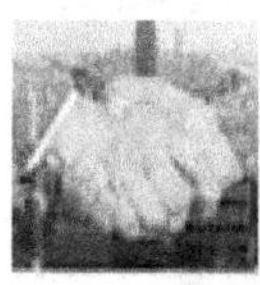

Conclusion

Table of Contents

Chapter 5: Understanding the Role of Habits 106

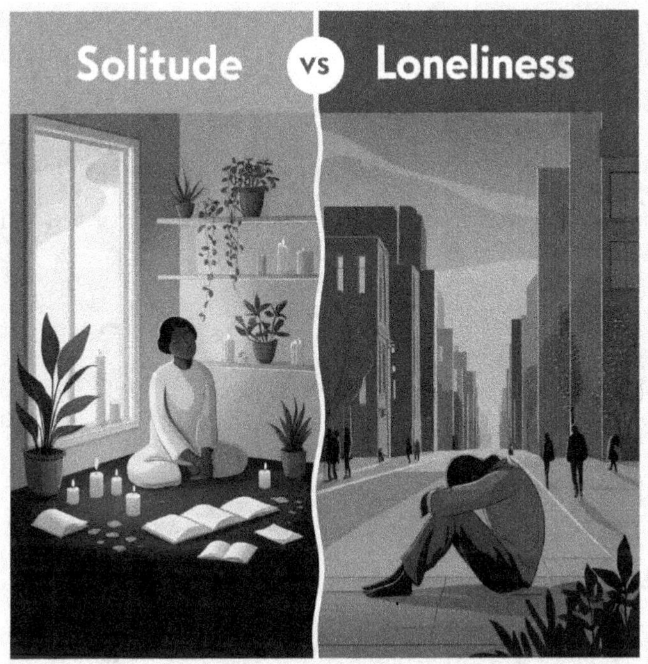

Chapter 1: Introduction to Solitude

The Difference Between "Solitude" and "Loneliness"

Have you ever been in a bustling café, surrounded by people laughing and chatting, yet felt an overwhelming sense of emptiness? It's a strange paradox, isn't it? This feeling perfectly illustrates the difference between being "alone" and feeling "lonely." Understanding this distinction is key as you begin your journey toward renewal, whereas "aloneness" is also called solitude.

Solitude: Aloneness

Aloneness, also called solitude, is simply the state of being by yourself. But here's the important part—it doesn't have to feel lonely. In fact, being alone can be a deeply positive experience. It's a chance to reflect, explore your creativity, and grow in ways that aren't always possible when you're constantly surrounded by others. When you embrace aloneness, you create a space to reconnect with your inner self.

Emotional Impact of Aloneness

Spending time alone, in solitude, can lead to feelings of contentment, peace, and even empowerment. It gives you the opportunity to recharge, to step back, and engage in activities that reflect what you love and what matters to you. In these moments, aloneness becomes something that energizes and nourishes you, rather than something to avoid.

Loneliness

In contrast to solitude, loneliness is an emotional state where you feel isolated, empty, and disconnected—even when you're surrounded by others. It often comes from unmet emotional needs or a deep longing for more meaningful connections. Loneliness isn't just about being physically alone; it's about feeling emotionally out of touch with those around you.

Emotional Impact of Loneliness

Loneliness can take a heavy toll. It's linked to feelings of anxiety, depression, and can lower your self-esteem. When you crave connection but don't feel it, loneliness can create a cycle of despair. The more you yearn for those connections, the more isolated you feel when they don't happen, deepening that sense of emptiness.

The Emotional Landscape

Understanding the emotional differences between solitude and loneliness is essential for personal growth. Let's break it down:

Quality of Experience:

This is a time for self-discovery, reflection, and relaxation. It's about embracing solitude in a way that rejuvenates you. <u>Aloneness</u>

On the other hand, loneliness can push you toward emotional escape, sometimes through unhealthy habits like overindulgence or avoidance. Loneliness

Independence vs. Dependence.

Fosters a sense of independence and self-sufficiency. It's a way to build emotional resilience by learning to rely on yourself. <u>Aloneness.</u>

Often involves a longing for connection, which can lead to emotional dependence on others for validation and fulfillment. <u>Loneliness</u>

Mental Health Impact:

When embraced with a positive mindset, it can actually enhance your mental well-being, offering clarity and peace. <u>Aloneness.</u>

However, loneliness is linked to increased risks of mental health issues such as depression, anxiety, and chronic stress. <u>Loneliness</u>

The Impact of Loneliness

The longer you feel lonely, the harder it becomes to break free. Anxiety and depression can build up, and it becomes this cycle— feeling isolated makes you pull away from others, which only deepens that isolation. <u>Mental Health</u>: You might not realize it, but loneliness can affect your physical health too. Studies have found that loneliness can lead to heart problems and a weaker immune system, among other things. It's like your body reacts to that emotional isolation by breaking down. <u>Physical Health</u>

Loneliness can also affect your spiritual well-being. Over time, the sense of isolation can make you feel disconnected from your purpose or a deeper sense of meaning in life. This disconnection can lead to feelings of emptiness or even a crisis of faith, making it harder to find peace or fulfillment. <u>Spiritual Health</u>

The Benefits of Solitude on the Life

But here's the flip side: solitude. Unlike loneliness, solitude is something you can embrace. It's a time to be alone, sure, but it doesn't have to feel empty. Solitude can be a space for growth, self-reflection, and renewal. When you're alone, without the usual distractions, something interesting happens you start to listen to yourself. Time spent in solitude allows you to really reflect on your thoughts, your emotions, and the experiences you've had. It's through this kind of introspection that you begin to understand yourself better. You see what drives you, what makes you happy, and even what might be holding you back. <u>Self-Reflection</u>

You know, there's a reason why so many artists, writers, and creative minds turn to solitude for inspiration. It is rewarding. When you're not caught up in social interactions or the demands of everyday life, your mind has the freedom to wander. It's in this quiet space that new ideas often come to life. Without those constant distractions, you start to think more deeply and creatively—solitude can be like fuel for your imagination. <u>Creativity Boost</u>

Learning to be comfortable with being alone is a huge step in building emotional strength. When you're okay with solitude, it means you've learned how to rely on yourself for happiness and fulfillment. You stop needing others to validate your worth, and instead, you find that strength within. This kind of resilience is incredibly empowering; it helps you weather life's ups and downs without constantly needing external reassurance. <u>Emotional Resilience</u>

Solitude is the perfect setting for mindfulness. Whether it's through meditation or just sitting quietly with your thoughts, being alone allows you to slow down. It gives you the space to become more aware of what's going on inside your mind and body. The result? Less stress, more clarity, and an overall sense of calm. Even just a few minutes of mindful solitude can make a big difference. <u>Mindfulness Practice</u>

I remember a time when I experienced a profound shift during a weekend spent alone. No plans, no distractions, just me. I took a long walk through a quiet remote field, and somewhere along the path, I found clarity about a decision I'd been struggling with for months. It was as if the solitude gave me the mental space to hear my own voice more clearly, to understand what I truly wanted. Those moments of quiet reflection can be incredibly powerful.

Please! Now, take a moment to think about solitude in your own life.

What does solitude mean to you?

Can you recall a time when being alone helped you gain clarity or a deeper understanding of something important?

CALL TO ACTION

Over the next week, I invite you to commit to just 10 minutes a day of solitude. Find a quiet space, free from distractions, and simply be with your thoughts. Use this time to reflect, to think, or just to breathe.

Understanding the difference between loneliness and solitude is crucial to starting this journey toward renewal. When you embrace the benefits of solitude, you change the way you experience being alone. It becomes less about discomfort and more about growth. This shift can be transformative, turning solitude into one of your most powerful tools for personal development.

Identifying the Problem

Do you ever feel like you're juggling too many things at once, and no matter how hard you try, you can't keep up? Life can often feel like a balancing act, especially when the physical, mental, and spiritual sides of yourself aren't in sync. This kind of imbalance can leave you feeling scattered, exhausted, and uncertain about where to turn next. Recognizing these issues is the first step toward getting your focus and sense of well-being back. Imbalances in Life

Mental Factors Contributing to Imbalance

Between the constant flood of emails, notifications, and social media updates, it's no surprise that mental exhaustion sets in. With so much information thrown at you, focusing on what really matters gets tough. Overwhelm from Information Overload

When stress levels are through the roof, your mind is too busy worrying to focus on anything else. Mental fatigue kicks in, and suddenly, even the simplest tasks feel overwhelming. It's hard to enjoy peaceful moments when your mind is always racing. Stress and Anxiety

Without practicing mindfulness, you might find yourself disconnected from the present. Instead of being fully in the moment, your thoughts are scattered, leaving you feeling anxious and ungrounded. Lack of Mindfulness

Physical Factors Contributing to Imbalance

In a world that revolves around screens, it's easy to find yourself sitting for hours on end. The problem? All that sitting can lead to aches, fatigue, and even weight gain. Over time, your body starts to feel the strain, and it can drag you down in other areas of life too. Sedentary Lifestyle

Ever notice how your energy and mood dip after a day of eating junk food? What you put into your body has a huge impact on how you feel. When you're not getting the right nutrients, staying focused and energized becomes an uphill battle. Poor Nutrition

We've all had those nights where sleep just doesn't come, and the next day feels like a fog. Lack of sleep can seriously mess with your mind, making it harder to think clearly and handle stress. Without enough rest, it's no wonder life starts to feel off balance. Inadequate Sleep

Spiritual Factors Contributing to Imbalance

When your day-to-day life doesn't line up with what you truly believe or value, something feels off. It creates a kind of emptiness, as though you're going through the motions but not really feeling fulfilled. This spiritual disconnect can leave you wondering if you're on the right path. Disconnection from Values

It's easy to get caught up in everything else and forget to take care of yourself. But when you ignore self-care—whether it's through reflection or spiritual practices—you can start feeling burned out, lost, and unsure of where to find fulfillment. Neglecting Self-Care:

Work-Life Imbalance

In today's work culture, being busy is often worn like a badge of honor. But that constant hustle can take a toll. Many of us end up prioritizing work at the expense of our personal lives, and the results can be tough—strained relationships, decreased satisfaction in our jobs, and eventually, burnout. It's hard to feel balanced when work is always at the top of the list.

Emotional Overload

Juggling emotions can feel like a full-time job in itself. Whether it's stress from work, the pressures of family life, or social obligations, constantly managing those feelings can wear you out. Emotional exhaustion makes it difficult to find joy or clarity in everyday moments because you're always carrying the weight of those feelings with you.

Social Disconnection

It's strange! technology has made it easier than ever to stay connected, yet so many of us feel more isolated than ever. A big part of this is that a lot of our interactions have moved online, where connections can often feel shallow. Sure, we may be "talking" more, but without depth or real engagement, it's easy to feel socially disconnected.

I remember a time when I was completely caught up in work commitments and endless social obligations. I was always surrounded by people at gatherings, but despite being in a room full of friends, I felt incredibly isolated. It wasn't until I made the conscious decision to step back and spend some time alone that I began to reconnect with who I really was. That's when things finally started to fall back into place.

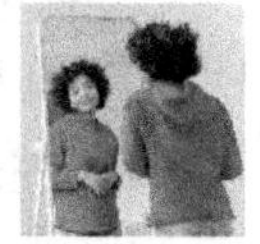

Now, take a moment to reflect on your own life:

Which areas feel scattered or out of balance?

Can you pinpoint specific physical, mental, or spiritual factors that might be contributing to that imbalance?

Over the next week, I encourage you to start a journal where you track moments when you feel scattered or overwhelmed. Try to identify the triggers that lead to these feelings and look for any patterns that emerge. This simple exercise can offer powerful insights into what's pulling you in too many directions. The accompanying resources—**a Planner**, <u>The 40-Day Solitude Planner </u>(Available at amazon KDP) and **a Notion Template**, <u>40 Days of Clarity </u>(available at gumroad.com),

Understanding what causes scattering and imbalance is the first step in your journey toward renewal. Once you can see the factors at play, you're in a better position to take meaningful steps toward living a more focused and fulfilling life. This section has laid out some clear concepts to help you begin, and with personal stories, reflection prompts, and actionable steps, you're now ready to dive deeper into the work ahead.

Presenting the Solution

Have you ever wished for a guide to help you navigate through the chaos of life? Imagine a path that offers clarity, insight, and a stronger connection to yourself with each passing day. That's what the **40-Day Guide to Solitude and Renewal** is all about—a structured framework designed to help you regain balance, focus, and a sense of well-being.

The 40-Day Framework: Overview of the Journey

This guide is built on three core pillars: <u>Physical Renewal, Mental Improvement, and Spiritual Growth.</u> Each week focuses on one of these pillars, giving you the time and space to fully engage with practices that will transform your life, one day at a time.

Week 1: Physical Renewal

The first week is all about laying the foundation for a healthier body and lifestyle. You'll focus on establishing daily routines that prioritize your physical well-being. This includes incorporating exercise and making sure you're getting enough rest—both of which are key to setting yourself up for success.

Week 2: Mental Improvement

Once your physical foundation is set, the second week shifts toward the mind. Here, you'll dive into mindfulness practices, explore ways to engage in lifelong learning, and focus on building emotional resilience. It's about training your mind to handle challenges with clarity and strength.

Week 3: Spiritual Growth

In the third week, your focus shifts to nurturing your spiritual self. This is a time to explore spiritual practices that resonate with you, whether through meditation, prayer, or something else that feeds your soul. Take time to connect with nature, as it offers a powerful way to find grounding and clarity. You'll also focus on serving others, recognizing that spiritual growth often involves giving back in meaningful ways.

Week 4-6: Integration and Reflection

Week 4-6. Tree weeks, are all about tying everything together. You'll reflect on your entire journey, integrating the changes you've made into your daily routine so that they stick long after the 40 days are over. This is your chance to set new goals for continued growth, ensuring that the work you've done doesn't end here but becomes a lasting part of your life.

Daily Structure

Here's what each day will look like:

Start your day by setting intentions that align with your goals, whether it's focusing on your physical health, mental clarity, or spiritual growth. <u>Morning Intentions</u>

You'll engage in specific exercises or activities that are tied to the theme of the week. These practices will help you build strength, resilience, and insight. <u>Daily Practices</u>

Before you end your day, take a moment to reflect on what you learned, how you felt, and what progress you've made. <u>Evening Reflections:</u>

Interactive Elements

At the end of each week, you'll find tools to help you track your journey and stay on course:

Questions that encourage you to think about your progress and the insights you've gained during the week.

Action Steps: Practical tasks designed to reinforce what you've learned and to keep the momentum going, even as you move forward.

I remember when I first started this framework myself. During the first week, when I was focused on physical renewal, I really struggled to stick to my new exercise routine. Every day felt like a challenge. But by the end of that week, I started noticing something—my energy levels were higher, and I felt stronger, not just physically, but mentally too. That's when I realized this was more than just a physical change—it was the beginning of something much deeper.

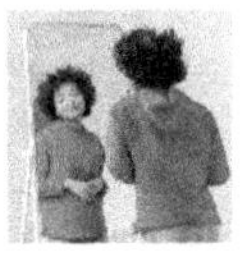

Before you set out on this journey of solitude and renewal, take a moment to think about your intentions. What is it that you hope to achieve over the next 40 days? Jot down your goals—whether it's finding balance, gaining clarity, or nurturing your physical, mental, or spiritual self. Keep those goals in sight as a reminder of your commitment to the process.

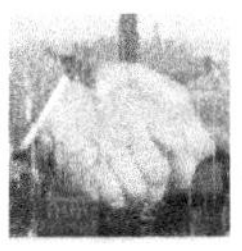

Ask yourself these questions as you prepare:

What parts of your life feel the most unbalanced right now?

How do you see solitude helping you in this renewal process?

The <u>40-Day Guide to Solitude and Renewal</u> isn't just another plan—it's an invitation to step away from the constant noise of everyday life and reconnect with yourself. By committing to this journey, you're opening the door to resilience, clarity, and a deeper understanding of who you are. This section not only introduces the framework for the journey but also encourages you to dive in with personal reflection, actionable steps, and insights that can transform your life.

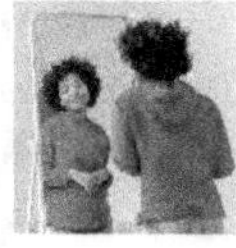

I remember one weekend when I found myself alone in my apartment, and at first, I dreaded the idea. The silence felt overwhelming, and I wasn't sure how I'd fill the time. But as the hours passed, something shifted. I began to embrace the quiet—watching movies I'd been meaning to see, reading books, and taking time to journal my thoughts. What surprised me the most was the sense of peace that gradually took over. By the end of the weekend, I realized that being alone wasn't something to fear. In fact, it was something beautiful, a chance to reconnect with myself in a way I hadn't done in years. That experience changed my entire outlook on solitude, turning it into something empowering rather than isolating.

Take a moment to reflect:

How do you feel when you're by yourself?

Can you recall times when you've felt lonely, even when you were surrounded by others?

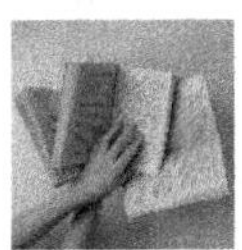

For the next week, pay close attention to your emotions during moments of solitude. Try journaling about how you feel. Do you experience empowerment and peace, or do you lean more toward feelings of loneliness? Use these insights as a foundation for the journey you're about to embark on.

Understanding the difference between aloneness and loneliness is crucial as you begin this transformative journey. By choosing to embrace aloneness as an opportunity for personal growth, rather than fearing loneliness, you open the door to a deeper understanding of who you are and what you need. This shift in perspective can be life-changing.

Finding Peace in Aloneness

Last year, I made a decision that felt both exciting and a little daunting—I planned a solo weekend retreat in a cozy cabin, tucked away deep in the woods. As I drove farther from the city, I couldn't help but wonder: would the quiet be overwhelming? Would I find myself missing the company of my friends? There was a part of me that wasn't quite sure how I'd handle the solitude.

Experience of Aloneness

When I finally arrived, nature greeted me with open arms. The gentle rustling of leaves, the chorus of chirping birds, and the soft gurgle of a nearby stream created a peaceful backdrop. After unpacking, I felt something I hadn't experienced in a long time—a wave of calm settled over me. For the first time in what felt like ages, I was completely alone. No buzzing phone, no meetings or social gatherings, just me and my thoughts. That evening, I prepared a simple meal and savoured every bite as the sun dipped below the trees. As night fell, I curled up by the fireplace with a book, feeling more at ease than I had in a long while. In that quiet moment, I realized that being alone wasn't the same as being lonely. Instead, it was a rare opportunity to really sit with my thoughts and feelings without any outside noise.

Transition to Loneliness

But as the night grew darker and the stillness deepened, something shifted. The silence that had been so comforting during the day started to feel a little heavier. I found myself longing for someone to share the moment with—whether it was laughing over dinner or chatting about the book I was reading. That quiet ache of loneliness began to creep in, making me hyper-aware of my solitude.

Resolution

The next morning, I decided to take a long hike through the woods, letting each step guide my thoughts. As I walked, I reflected on the loneliness I'd felt the night before. I began to realize that, while loneliness was a reminder of what I didn't have, aloneness had given me something just as valuable—an opportunity for self-discovery. By leaning into both emotions, I started to see solitude not as something to escape but as a space to grow and find clarity.

When I returned home, I didn't just carry memories of peaceful moments in the woods—I brought back a deeper understanding of myself. That weekend alone gave me strength and clarity, and even the loneliness had taught me something important: the value of connection and the beauty of aloneness, side by side.

This experience taught me something important: while loneliness can feel isolating and even painful at times, aloneness can be deeply enriching and transformative. Both states—loneliness and aloneness—are part of being human. But the real difference lies in how we navigate them. It's through our approach to solitude that we shape our personal journey and growth. This story highlights the contrast between aloneness as a positive, reflective space and loneliness as a yearning for connection. It's a reminder that personal growth often comes through embracing solitude.

Setting Expectations for Transformation

What if, in just 40 days, you could completely transform your relationship with yourself and the world around you? Picture waking up every day feeling more grounded, focused, and connected to who you truly are. This journey isn't just about spending time alone—it's about rediscovering yourself and finding out what really matters to you.

Attaining Solitude in a Busy Life: Integrating Renewal into Work and Daily Responsibilities

Solitude doesn't always mean stepping away from all responsibilities or retreating into complete isolation. In fact, solitude can be practiced right within your busy workday, business environment, or daily routines. By cultivating small but intentional moments of solitude, you can find ways to renew and ground yourself, even amidst a packed schedule. Here, we'll explore several methods for integrating solitude into various aspects of a busy life.

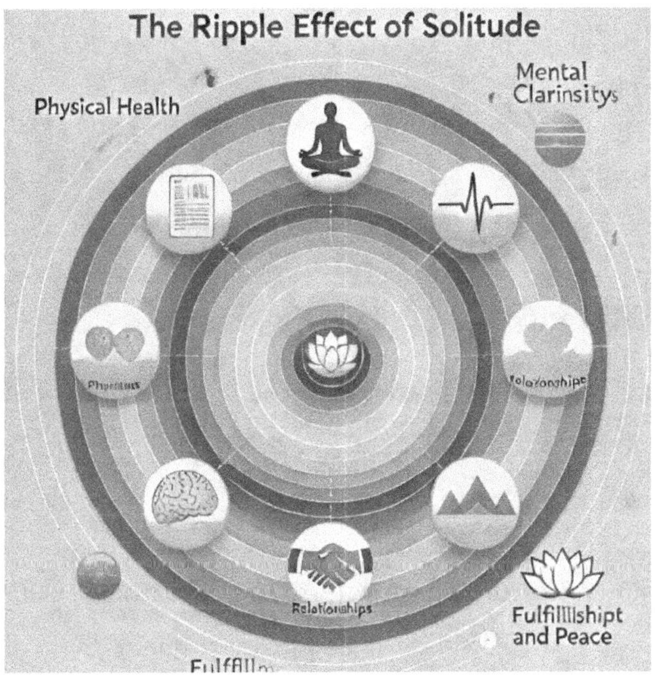

1. Mindful Transitions Between Tasks

Often, we move from one task to another without pause, which can leave us feeling exhausted or scattered. A moment of intentional solitude between tasks can help you reset your mind, fostering clarity and focus.

Practice: Before starting a new task, take a minute or two to close your eyes, take a few deep breaths, and release any tension. Try to focus on your breathing, and clear your mind of any leftover thoughts from the previous task.

Benefit: This practice serves as a mental "reset button," helping you enter the next task with fresh energy and a calm mind.

2. Creating "Micro-Retreats" in Your Workspace

Designing small, intentional spaces within your work environment can create moments of solitude that allow you to recharge without leaving the office.

Practice: Dedicate a corner of your desk, or find a nearby quiet space, where you can take short "micro-retreats" during the day. Use this space for brief meditation, journaling, or even a few moments of silence.

Benefit: This can create a sense of personal sanctuary amidst the busyness, giving you a space to unwind and reconnect with yourself whenever needed.

3. Scheduling Solitude Breaks

Incorporating solitude into your daily routine can be as simple as scheduling it, just as you would any other work meeting or appointment. Even a few minutes of undisturbed time can foster renewal.

Practice: Block out short periods in your schedule where you'll be free from interruptions—such as stepping outside, finding a quiet room, or even staying at your desk with headphones on to discourage conversation.

Benefit: Regular solitude breaks can help you manage stress, prevent burnout, and enhance creativity and focus throughout the day.

4. Practicing Solitude During Commutes

Commutes, whether by car, bus, or train, offer a hidden opportunity for solitude if approached with intention. Rather than filling this time with calls, emails, or constant media consumption, use it as a chance to center yourself.

Practice: Try spending part of your commute in silence, using this time to practice mindful breathing, observe the scenery, or simply be present. Avoid checking your phone or planning your day; instead, let this be a pocket of solitude within your routine.

Benefit: Using your commute for solitude can bring a sense of calm and grounding, preparing you to start or end the day with a refreshed mind.

5. Solitude Through Intentional Digital Boundaries

Our constant connectivity can erode any chance for solitude, making it vital to set boundaries around digital communication and device usage. Creating intentional tech-free times during the day can foster solitude even within busy schedules.

Practice: Designate specific times to turn off notifications, step away from screens, or place your phone on "Do Not Disturb" mode. This might be during meals, for an hour each morning, or right before bed.

Benefit: By disconnecting from digital demands, you're able to enter a space of solitude, giving yourself the opportunity to recharge and reflect without constant distractions.

6. Solitude Through Reflection and End-of-Day Rituals

Ending the day with moments of solitude can help you wind down, reflect on the day's events, and prepare for a restful night.

This can be a grounding practice, especially if the day has been filled with constant activity.

Practice: Dedicate a few minutes each evening to sit quietly, journal, or review the day's achievements and challenges. Reflect on any moments you felt present and any insights you gained about yourself.

Benefit: A reflective end-of-day ritual can help you integrate solitude into your daily routine, supporting mental clarity, emotional balance, and restful sleep.

40-Day Plan: A Six-Week Journey to Physical, Mental, and Spiritual Renewal

This 40-day plan is structured to build momentum gradually, introducing changes that feel manageable while offering powerful benefits. Each week focuses on one or more aspects of wellness—physical, mental, and spiritual—so that by the end, you'll have integrated habits that nurture every part of yourself. The first three weeks emphasize introducing and layering new practices, while the final three weeks focus on deepening and solidifying these habits into a sustainable, enjoyable routine. Let's break   down   how   this   journey   unfolds.

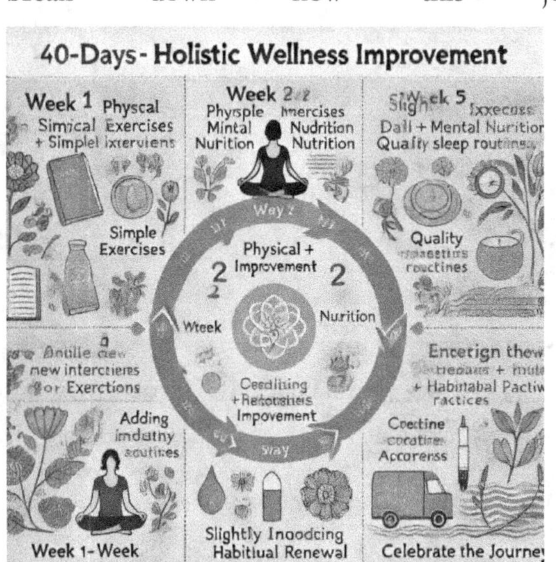

Week 1: Laying the Foundation – Physical Improvement

The journey begins with a focus on the physical body, which is often the most tangible place to start. By prioritizing physical improvement first, you'll begin to feel more energized and resilient, which can have a positive effect on mental clarity and emotional well-being. The practices in Week 1 are designed to be approachable and enjoyable, helping you ease into the habit of self-care.

Daily Movement: Start with simple forms of exercise like walking, stretching, or light strength exercises. Each day includes a

15–20-minute physical activity session, with an emphasis on consistency rather than intensity.

Hydration and Nutrition: Incorporate more water and nutrient-dense foods into your diet. Focus on small adjustments, like drinking a glass of water first thing in the morning and adding a serving of vegetables to each meal.

Rest and Recovery: Prioritize sleep this week by creating a bedtime routine. Set a consistent time to wind down, avoiding screens and incorporating relaxation techniques to promote restful sleep.

By the end of Week 1, you'll likely feel an increase in energy and vitality, setting the stage for further growth.

Week 2: Building on the Physical with Mental Improvement

In Week 2, the focus expands to include mental wellness alongside physical practices. This week is about cultivating mindfulness and enhancing mental clarity. Adding mental practices helps you stay engaged with the physical improvements from Week 1 while introducing exercises to foster calmness and focus.

Mindfulness Exercises: Begin each day with a few minutes of deep breathing or a quick meditation session. This could involve simple breath awareness, body scanning, or guided mindfulness exercises to ground you before the day starts.

Reflective Journaling: Each day, take 5–10 minutes to journal about your thoughts, goals, or any mental patterns you notice. This practice will enhance self-awareness and help release any stress or mental clutter that may arise.

Continued Physical Routine: Maintain the physical routines from Week 1—movement, hydration, and rest—while now including moments of mindfulness throughout the day.

This week integrates the mind with the body, creating a foundation of awareness and calm that will support you as you continue.

Week 3: Adding Spiritual Improvement

Week 3 brings a deeper focus on spiritual well-being. Spiritual improvement in this plan is about connecting with your inner self, exploring purpose, and finding meaning. Integrating spiritual practices with your physical and mental routines allows you to nurture a sense of purpose, inner peace, and connection.

Daily Reflection or Meditation: Begin each day with a reflective question or meditation that invites you to explore your inner values, purpose, and gratitude. Examples might include "What am I grateful for?" or "What impact do I want to have on others today?"

Affirmations and Intentions: Write and repeat a positive affirmation or intention daily to keep you centered. This could be as simple as "I am open to growth" or "I am connected to my purpose."

Nature and Silence: Spend a few minutes each day in nature or in silence, practicing presence and embracing a sense of oneness with your surroundings. This can foster feelings of connection and tranquillity.

Continued Physical and Mental Practices: Keep up with the physical and mental routines from previous weeks, strengthening these habits while introducing spiritual renewal.

At the end of Week 3, you should feel a growing sense of balance across all three domains—physical, mental, and spiritual.

Weeks 4–6: Deepening, Integrating, and Creating Consistency

The final three weeks are focused on consistency, enjoyment, and creating a sustainable, balanced routine. By now, the foundation has been laid for a holistic approach to wellness, and these weeks are about strengthening the habits developed. These weeks emphasize integrating these practices seamlessly into your life, solidifying them into enjoyable routines that you'll look forward to each day.

Week 4: Deepening the Habits

Week 4 is about making these practices feel like a natural part of your day. You'll continue to follow the physical, mental, and spiritual practices, but with an emphasis on deepening each one to explore new dimensions of growth.

Increasing Intensity or Duration: Slightly increase the intensity or duration of your physical exercises, mindful practices, or meditation to build strength and resilience.

Personal Reflection: Set aside time to assess the progress you've made, what you've found enjoyable, and areas that may need adjustment. This is also a time to celebrate small wins and continue with what's working.

Accountability Check: To enhance consistency, consider sharing your progress with a friend or journaling about your experiences. Accountability can reinforce your commitment.

Week 5: Adding Variety and Fun

During Week 5, you'll introduce variety to keep the routine fresh and engaging. This is the time to experiment with new activities or variations of your practices to make the journey enjoyable and stimulating.

Explore New Forms of Exercise or Mindfulness: Try a new form of exercise or mindfulness practice, like a different type of yoga, tai chi, or creative expression such as drawing or dancing.

Connect with Others: Find a like-minded community, whether online or offline, to share insights and engage in discussions about wellness. If you've joined the Telegram channel for this book, share your journey and learn from others.

Mindful Creativity: Engage in creative or artistic activities, allowing yourself to express ideas and emotions freely. This can be a meditative, rejuvenating practice that enhances both mental and spiritual growth.

Week 6: Cultivating Habitual Renewal

The final week is about reinforcing everything you've learned, turning these practices into lifelong habits. By now, you'll have a clear understanding of what practices resonate with you most and how they contribute to a sense of renewal.

Solidifying Daily Routines: Make a commitment to incorporate the practices that resonate most, whether that's daily movement, mindful moments, or evening reflection.

Developing a Sustainable Schedule: Set realistic goals for maintaining these practices beyond the program. Consider how often you'll incorporate each habit, and let it be adaptable to fit your life going forward.

Reflect and Celebrate: Reflect on your journey over the past 40 days, acknowledging the growth and progress made. Celebrate these accomplishments, knowing they have prepared you for sustainable, balanced wellness.

Potential Outcomes of Your Journey

1. Enhanced Self-Awareness

By spending time in solitude, you'll gain deeper insights into your own thoughts, emotions, and behaviors. This self-awareness will help you make more conscious choices that align with your values and long-term goals.

2. Improved Mental Clarity

As you commit to daily mindfulness practices, you'll start to notice a real shift—mental clutter begins to clear. This newfound clarity will help you focus on what truly matters, allowing you to become more productive and make better decisions in both your personal and professional life.

3. Greater Emotional Resilience

By facing feelings of loneliness head-on and learning to embrace aloneness, you'll build emotional strength. This resilience will equip you to handle life's challenges with more confidence and grace, no longer relying on external factors for emotional stability.

4. Deeper Connections

The more comfortable you become in your own company, the more your relationships with others will flourish. You'll notice that you're able to engage with friends, family, and colleagues in more authentic and meaningful ways. Being at peace with yourself will allow you to connect with others on a deeper level.

5. A Renewed Sense of Purpose

This journey is also about reconnecting with what drives you. As you spend time reflecting, you may uncover new passions or reignite old dreams that had been set aside. By the end of the 40 days, you could find yourself setting new goals or rediscovering long-lost interests that fill your life with joy and fulfillment.

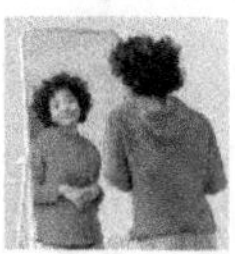

I remember when I first embarked on a journey like this. At the start, I was hesitant—unsure of how I'd handle the time alone. But as the days passed, I found myself reflecting deeply on the direction my life was headed. By the end of those weeks, not only did I gain clarity about my career, but I also reignited a passion for painting—something I hadn't done in years. The transformation was remarkable; it reminded me that solitude isn't just about being alone, it can be a powerful catalyst for rediscovering yourself.

Take a moment to reflect:

What specific changes do you hope to see in yourself by the end of this journey?

How do you imagine solitude playing a role in creating those changes?

CALL TO ACTION

Before moving forward, write down three intentions you want to focus on during this journey. What do you hope to achieve over the next 40 days? Keep these intentions somewhere visible to remind you of your commitment to personal transformation.

Setting clear expectations for transformation is a key part of starting this journey of solitude and renewal. When you embrace this process with an open heart and mind, you create space for profound changes to unfold in your life.

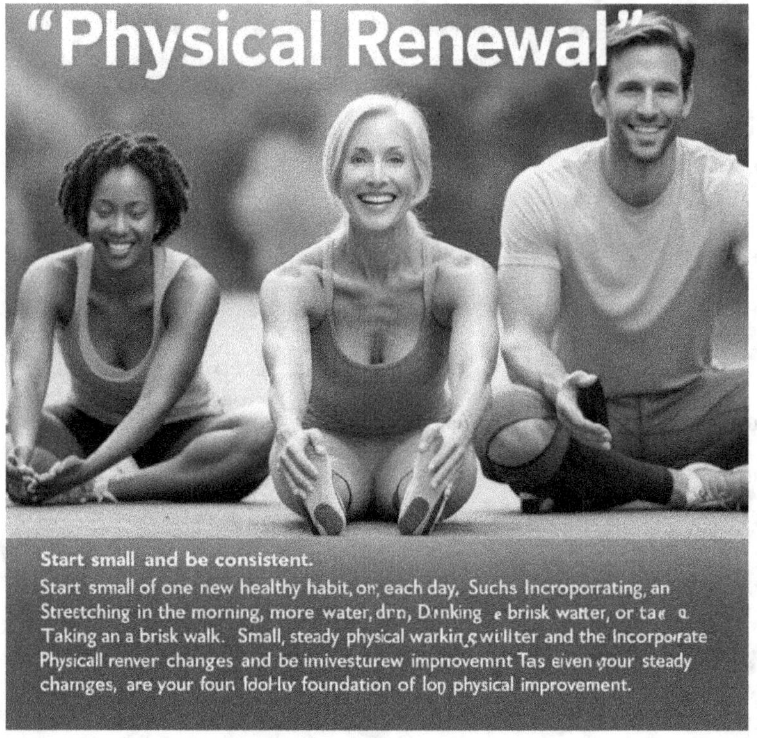

Chapter 2: Physical Renewal

Establishing a Healthy Routine

Have you ever felt like the day just slips away, leaving little time for yourself? If so, you're not alone. Creating a balanced daily routine is essential for both physical renewal and your overall sense of well-being. By intentionally structuring your day, you can make your health and happiness a priority, rather than an afterthought.

Creating a Balanced Daily Schedule

1. Start with a Morning Ritual

Kickstart your day with a routine that sets a positive tone. Here are a few simple practices to consider: Drink a glass of water as soon as you wake up to jump start your metabolism and hydrate your body. <u>Hydration.</u> Engage in some light stretching or a quick workout to get your body moving and boost your energy for the day. <u>Movement.</u> Spend a few minutes meditating or journaling to centre your thoughts and set a calm, focused mindset for the day ahead. <u>Mindfulness.</u>

2. Prioritize Nutrition

Fuelling your body with the right foods is essential for maintaining energy and focus. Here are some tips for making nutrition a priority: Set aside some time each week to prepare healthy meals and snacks, so you have nutritious options ready when you're busy. <u>Meal Prep</u>. Take time to enjoy your meals without distractions. Focus on the flavors, textures, and the act of nourishing your body. <u>Mindful Eating</u>

3. Schedule Regular Exercise

Physical activity is key to maintaining your energy and well-being. Incorporate exercise into your routine with these strategies:

Treat your workouts like important appointments. Block out specific times on your calendar and stick to them. <u>Set Specific Times</u>. Keep things interesting by trying different forms of exercise—whether it's yoga, running, dancing, or something new. Variety keeps it enjoyable and prevents burnout. <u>Mix It Up.</u>

4. Create Breaks for Rest

Prevent burnout by scheduling regular breaks to recharge: Try working in 25-minute intervals, followed by a 5-minute break. This method helps maintain focus and energy throughout the day. <u>Pomodoro Technique</u>. Step outside for a breath of fresh air and sunlight, even if it's just for a few minutes. These small moments of connection with nature can be incredibly refreshing. <u>Nature Breaks.</u>

5. Wind Down in the Evening

Create an evening routine that helps you relax and prepare for restful sleep:

Turn off your devices at least an hour before bed to improve the quality of your sleep. <u>Limit Screen Time</u>. Take a few moments to journal about what went well or what you're grateful for. This simple reflection can bring a sense of closure to your day and set a positive tone for tomorrow. <u>Reflect on Your Day</u>.

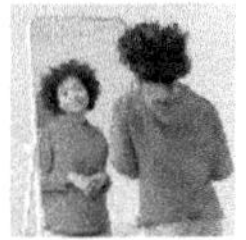

When I first started focusing on my physical renewal, finding time for exercise felt like an uphill battle. My schedule was packed, and squeezing in a workout seemed impossible. Then one day, I decided to wake up just 30 minutes earlier. That small change opened up space for a morning workout routine, and it completely transformed my energy levels throughout the day. It's amazing how a tiny adjustment can make such a big impact!

Take a moment to reflect on your own routine:

What does your typical day look like right now?

Where can you make small adjustments to prioritize your physical health?

Challenge yourself to create a balanced daily schedule based on the tips provided. Try to incorporate at least three new practices into your routine, and take note of how they affect your energy, mood, and overall well-being.

Building a healthy routine is the foundation for physical renewal. When you intentionally structure your day, you create the space for self-care and rejuvenation, setting the stage for deeper transformation throughout your journey.

Incorporating Regular Exercise

Have you ever started a new workout routine full of enthusiasm, only to watch that motivation fade after a few weeks? You're not alone sticking to regular exercise can be tough. But it's a key part of physical renewal and overall well-being. Let's dive into different types of exercises you can try, along with strategies to keep you motivated on your fitness journey.

Types of Exercises to Include

1. Cardiovascular Exercises

Cardio activities get your heart pumping and improve cardiovascular health. Here are a few options to get you moving:

Perfect for building endurance, and you can do it anywhere—outside or on a treadmill. <u>Running or Jogging</u>. A low-impact option that's gentle on your joints but great for your heart and legs. <u>Cycling</u>. Fun, energetic, and mood-lifting—dancing not only gets your heart rate up but also puts a smile on your face. <u>Dancing</u>.

2. Strength Training

Building muscle strength is essential for overall fitness. Here are some options to consider:

Push-ups, squats, and lunges don't require any equipment, so you can do them anywhere. <u>Bodyweight Exercises</u>. Whether using free weights or resistance machines, weightlifting helps you build muscle strength and tone your body. <u>Weightlifting</u>. These practices not only enhance flexibility but also build strength, making them great for both your body and mind. <u>Yoga or Pilates</u>.

3. Flexibility and Balance

Improving flexibility and balance is key to preventing injuries and boosting overall performance:

Make time to stretch your major muscle groups after each workout to keep your muscles healthy and limber. <u>Stretching.</u> A gentle, flowing martial art that helps with balance, flexibility, and relaxation—all while calming your mind. <u>Tai Chi.</u>

How to Stay Motivated

1. Set Realistic Goals

Start with goals that are manageable and gradually push yourself as you progress. For example, begin by walking for 15 minutes a day, then slowly work up to 30 minutes. Small, achievable goals can build confidence and keep you motivated to keep going.

2. Find an Accountability Partner

Exercising with a friend or joining a group class can make a world of difference. Not only does it add a fun social element, but it also helps keep you accountable. You're far less likely to skip a workout when someone else is counting on you to show up!

3. Mix It Up

Variety is key to keeping things exciting! Try alternating between different types of exercises throughout the week—this will prevent boredom and keep you engaged. From yoga one day to cycling the next, mixing it up keeps things fresh and fun.

4. Track Your Progress

Logging your workouts in a journal or using a fitness app can be incredibly motivating. Watching your progress over time, whether it's increasing your endurance or lifting heavier weights, reminds you just how far you've come.

When I first started my fitness journey, I struggled to stay motivated. I decided to join a local dance class, thinking it would be a fun way to move. To my surprise, I found myself genuinely looking forward to each session! The combination of movement and music brought joy back into my routine and made staying active feel less like a chore. That experience taught me that finding joy in exercise is the key to staying committed.

Take a moment to think about your current exercise habits:

What types of exercise do you enjoy?

How can you incorporate more movement into your daily life?

This week, challenge yourself to try out two new types of exercises. Schedule them into your routine and pay attention to how they make you feel—not just physically, but mentally as well. Reflect on whether they bring more energy or improve your mood throughout the day.

Incorporating regular exercise is a key part of your physical renewal journey. By exploring different activities and using strategies to stay motivated, you'll build a routine that not only improves.

Prioritizing Rest and Recovery

Have you ever noticed how one good night's sleep can completely change how you feel the next day? It's amazing how much rest can refresh not only your body but also your mind and spirit. Prioritizing rest and recovery are essential for physical renewal, yet it's something we often overlook in our busy lives. Let's take a closer look at the importance of sleep and a few effective ways to relax and recharge.

The Importance of Sleep

1. Physical Health

Quality sleep is essential for maintaining good physical health. When you sleep, your body goes into repair mode—it builds muscle, heals tissues, and strengthens your immune system. Without enough rest, your body can't function at its best, leading to a range of health issues, including:

Sleep deprivation messes with the hormones that control your appetite, often leading to overeating and cravings for unhealthy foods. Weight Gain. Poor sleep patterns are linked to a higher risk of chronic conditions like heart disease, diabetes, and high blood pressure. Increased Risk of Chronic Illness.

2. Mental Clarity

Sleep is essential for keeping your mind sharp and focused. When you're well-rested, your brain performs better, allowing you to think more clearly, solve problems, and stay productive. On the flip side, not getting enough sleep can lead to:

A lack of sleep makes it harder for your brain to consolidate and store memories effectively. Impaired Memory.

Fatigue can significantly impact your ability to focus on tasks and make sound decisions. Decreased Concentration.

3. Emotional Well-Being

Sleep also plays a critical role in maintaining emotional balance. When you're well-rested, you're better equipped to manage stress and maintain a positive mindset. However, when sleep is lacking:

Sleep deprivation can heighten your emotional responses, making you more prone to irritability or mood swings. <u>Increased Irritability.</u>

Not getting enough sleep can intensify feelings of anxiety and even contribute to depression. <u>Higher Anxiety Levels.</u>

Relaxation Techniques

In addition to prioritizing quality sleep, adding relaxation techniques to your daily routine can further enhance recovery and improve your overall well-being. Here are a few to consider:

1. Mindfulness Meditation

Spending just a few minutes each day practicing mindfulness can work wonders for reducing stress and promoting relaxation. By focusing on your breath or engaging in guided meditations, you can center your thoughts and bring calm to both your mind and body.

2. Deep Breathing Exercises

Deep breathing is a simple yet powerful way to activate your body's relaxation response. Here's an easy exercise to try:

- ✓ Inhale deeply through your nose for a count of four.

- ✓ Hold your breath for a count of four.

- ✓ Exhale slowly through your mouth for a count of six.

- ✓ Repeat this cycle several times, allowing your body to relax with each breath.

3. Gentle Stretching or Yoga

Incorporating gentle stretching or yoga into your routine can help release built-up tension and promote relaxation. Dedicating a few minutes each evening to unwind with light stretches or a calming yoga session can work wonders for both your body and mind.

I used to underestimate the power of sleep—until I experienced a particularly exhausting week at work. After several nights of poor sleep, I felt irritable, unfocused, and drained. It wasn't until I made a conscious effort to get at least seven hours of quality sleep each night that I noticed a huge improvement. My mood lifted, and my productivity soared. That week taught me an important lesson: rest isn't a luxury—it's an absolute necessity for thriving.

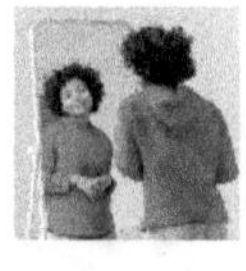

Take a moment to reflect on your current sleep habits:

How many hours of sleep do you typically get each night?

What relaxation techniques have you tried before bedtime?

Commit to establishing a bedtime routine that promotes quality sleep. Aim for at least seven hours of rest each night, and incorporate one relaxation technique into your evening routine.

Prioritizing rest and recovery is a crucial part of physical renewal. By understanding the importance of quality sleep and integrating effective relaxation techniques into your routine, you'll not only improve your physical health but also sharpen your mental clarity and boost your emotional well-being.

Week 1: Physical Improvement Reflection Prompts

In the following are daily reflection prompts aligned with the week 1, 40-day plan focusing on physical through solitude:

I'm excited to introduce my Notion template, <u>40 Days of Clarity</u> (available at gumroad.com), designed to enhance your reading experience. This template provides a structured way to organize your journey, allowing you to track your progress, set goals, and reflect on your insights as you navigate through the themes of solitude and self-discovery in the book.

Week 1: Physical Improvement

Day 1: Reflect on your current physical state. What improvements would you like to see in your health and fitness?

Day 2: Identify a physical activity that you enjoy. How can you incorporate it into your daily routine?

Day 3: Reflect on how your energy levels fluctuate during the day. What habits might help stabilize them?

Day 4: Consider your eating habits. What changes could support your physical well-being?

Day 5: Think about your sleep quality. What adjustments can you make for better rest?

Day 6: Reflect on any small physical victories you've experienced this week. How did they make you feel?

Day 7: Review the week. What changes in your physical well-being have you noticed?

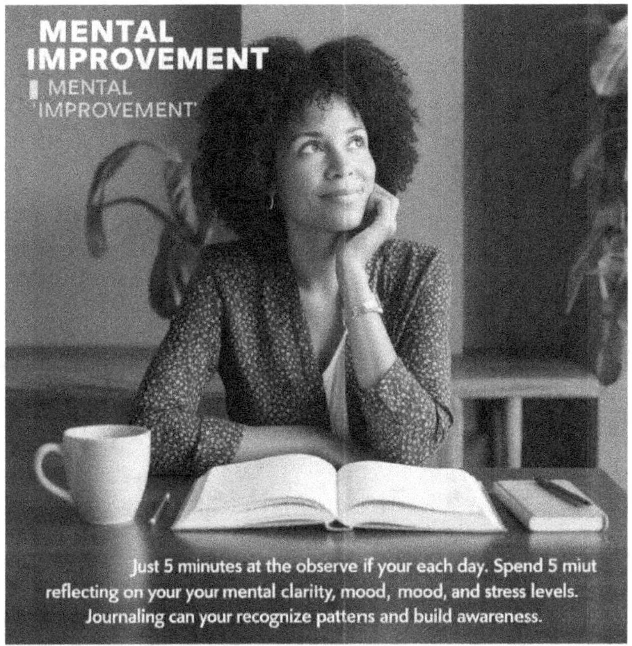

Chapter 3: Mental Improvement

Cultivating Mindfulness and Awareness

Have you ever gone through a day with your mind racing from task to task, barely taking a moment to pause and breathe? In today's fast-paced world, cultivating mindfulness can sometimes feel like a luxury. But it's essential for maintaining mental clarity and emotional balance. Let's dive into some simple mindfulness exercises that can easily fit into your daily routine.

The Importance of Mindfulness

Mindfulness is the practice of being fully present in the moment, engaging with your thoughts, feelings, and surroundings without judgment. This simple practice has countless benefits, including:

Practicing mindfulness lowers cortisol levels, helping you manage stress and reduce anxiety. <u>Reduced Stress.</u>

By staying present, mindfulness boosts your ability to concentrate on tasks and improve productivity. <u>Improved Focus.</u>

Mindfulness allows you to observe and acknowledge your emotions without being consumed by them, promoting a sense of balance. <u>Enhanced Emotional Regulation.</u>

Quick Mindfulness Exercises

1. Breathing Techniques

Breathing exercises are one of the simplest and most effective ways to cultivate mindfulness. Here are a couple of techniques you can try:

Deep Breathing:

✓ Find a comfortable seated position.

✓ Inhale deeply through your nose for a count of four.

✓ Hold your breath for a count of four.

✓ Exhale slowly through your mouth for a count of six.

✓ Repeat this cycle for several minutes, allowing your body to relax with each breath.

Box Breathing:

✓ Inhale through your nose for a count of four.

✓ Hold your breath for a count of four.

✓ Exhale through your mouth for a count of four.

✓ Hold again for a count of four.

✓ Repeat this process four times, noticing how your breath becomes steady and calming.

2. Body Scan Meditation

This mindfulness exercise helps you connect with your body and release any built-up tension:

✓ Lie down or sit comfortably in a quiet space.

✓ Close your eyes and take a few deep, calming breaths.

✓ Starting from your toes, slowly bring your awareness to each part of your body, moving upward.

✓ Pay attention to any sensations you feel—whether it's tension, relaxation, or discomfort—without judging or trying to change them. Simply observe and let go.

3. Mindful Walking

Walking can be a meditative experience if done mindfully:

✓ Find a quiet place where you can walk at a slow, comfortable pace.

✓ Focus on the sensation of your feet connecting with the ground with each step.

✓ Pay attention to the rhythm of your breathing as you walk.

✓ Engage with your surroundings by noticing the sounds, sights, and smells around you, while staying present in the moment

I remember the first time I tried mindfulness meditation. I sat cross-legged on my living room floor, determined to find peace in the silence. But after just a minute, my mind was racing with thoughts—dinner plans, work deadlines, and everything in between! It was frustrating at first, but with practice, I learned to gently bring my focus back to my breath each time my mind wandered. Over time, those brief moments of stillness became a sanctuary—a place where I could recharge and reconnect with myself.

Take a moment to reflect on your current mindfulness habits:

How often do you make time to truly be present in the moment?

What mindfulness techniques have you tried before, and how did they make you feel?

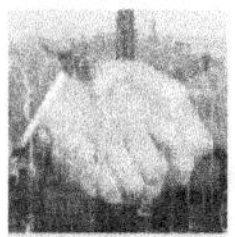

Pick one mindfulness exercise from the list above and commit to practicing it daily for at least five minutes. Pay attention to how it influences your mood and mental clarity throughout the day.

Cultivating mindfulness and awareness is essential for mental improvement and overall well-being. By incorporating these simple exercises into your daily routine, you can enhance your focus, reduce stress, and build a deeper connection with yourself.

Engaging in Lifelong Learning

Have you ever felt a spark of excitement when learning something new? That thrill of discovery can be one of life's greatest joys. Engaging in lifelong learning not only keeps your mind sharp but also enriches your life in countless ways. Let's explore how to set learning goals and dive into new interests that can transform your mental landscape.

The Importance of Lifelong Learning

Lifelong learning is the continuous, self-motivated pursuit of knowledge for personal or professional development. Here are some key benefits:

Regularly challenging your brain can improve memory and cognitive function. <u>Cognitive Health.</u>

In a rapidly changing world, being open to new knowledge helps you adapt to new situations and challenges. <u>Adaptability.</u>

Engaging in learning can lead to greater satisfaction and a sense of accomplishment. <u>Fulfillment.</u>

Setting Learning Goals

1. Identify Your Interests

Start by reflecting on what excites you. Consider:

- ✓ Hobbies you've always wanted to explore.

- ✓ Skills that could enhance your career.

- ✓ Topics you're passionate about but haven't had time to delve into.

2. Set SMART Goals

Use the SMART criteria to create effective learning goals:

Specific: Clearly define what you want to learn (e.g., "I want to learn basic Spanish").

Measurable: Determine how you will track your progress (e.g., "I will complete one lesson per week").

Achievable: Ensure your goal is realistic given your current commitments.

Relevant: Choose goals that align with your interests and aspirations.

Time-Bound: Set a deadline for achieving your goal (e.g., "I will be able to hold a basic conversation in three months").

3. Create a Learning Plan

Outline the steps needed to achieve your goals:

Identify resources such as books, online courses, or local classes.

Schedule regular time slots for learning in your calendar.

Exploring New Interests

1. Join a Class or Workshop

Participating in classes—whether online or in-person—can provide structure and community support. Look for workshops that align with your interests, such as cooking, art, or technology.

2. Read Widely

Reading is one of the best ways to expand your knowledge. Set a goal to read a certain number of books each month across various genres.

3. Engage with Online Resources

Platforms like Coursera, Udemy, or Khan Academy offer courses on a wide range of topics. Explore subjects that intrigue you and enroll in a course that fits your schedule.

When I decided to learn photography, I felt overwhelmed by the technical aspects. I set a goal to take one online course and practice taking photos every weekend. As I progressed, I discovered not just the mechanics of photography but also my passion for capturing moments in nature. This journey not only enhanced my skills but also provided me with a creative outlet that brought me immense joy.

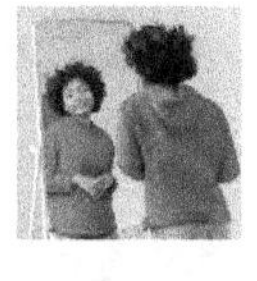

Take a moment to think about your own learning journey:

What new skills or knowledge would you like to acquire?

How can you incorporate lifelong learning into your daily routine?

Choose one new interest or skill you'd like to explore. Set a SMART goal around it and outline the steps you'll take to achieve it.

Engaging in lifelong learning is a powerful way to enhance mental improvement and enrich your life. By setting clear goals and exploring new interests, you'll not only expand your knowledge but also discover new passions along the way.

Building Emotional Resilience

Have you ever faced a challenge that felt insurmountable, only to emerge stronger on the other side? Building emotional resilience is like developing a muscle; it requires practice and dedication. In this section, we'll explore strategies to manage stress and enhance your emotional well-being, enabling you to bounce back from life's challenges.

The Importance of Emotional Resilience

Emotional resilience is the ability to adapt to stress and adversity. It's not about avoiding difficulties but rather learning how to navigate through them with strength and grace. Here are some key benefits:

Resilient individuals handle stress more effectively, reducing its impact on their mental health. <u>Improved Stress Management.</u>

Resilience fosters a proactive mindset, allowing you to approach challenges with creativity and confidence. <u>Enhanced Problem-Solving Skills.</u>

Building resilience leads to a more positive outlook on life, increasing overall happiness and fulfillment. <u>Greater Life Satisfaction.</u>

Strategies to Manage Stress

1. Practice Deep Breathing

Deep breathing is a simple yet powerful technique to calm your mind and body. Here's how:

Sit comfortably with your hands in your lap.

Close your eyes and take a deep breath in through your nose for a count of four.

Hold your breath for a count of four.

Exhale slowly through your mouth for a count of six.

Repeat this for 5–10 minutes whenever you feel stressed.

2. Engage in Regular Exercise

Physical activity is one of the most effective ways to combat stress. Aim for at least 30 minutes of moderate exercise most days of the week. Whether it's walking, dancing, or yoga, find an activity you enjoy!

3. Establish a Support Network

Connecting with others can provide emotional support during tough times:

Reach out to friends or family when you're feeling overwhelmed.

Consider joining a support group or community organization to meet new people.

4. Set Boundaries

Learn to say no to requests that overwhelm you. Setting limits helps protect your time and energy, allowing you to focus on what truly matters.

5. Practice Mindfulness

Incorporating mindfulness practices into your daily routine can enhance emotional resilience:

Spend a few minutes each day meditating or practicing gratitude.

Take time to reflect on positive experiences or things you're grateful for.

I remember a particularly stressful period at work when deadlines were piling up. I felt overwhelmed and anxious until I decided to take control by implementing deep breathing exercises during my breaks. These moments of calm allowed me to refocus my energy and tackle my tasks more effectively. Over time, I learned that building resilience isn't just about enduring challenges; it's about equipping myself with tools to thrive.

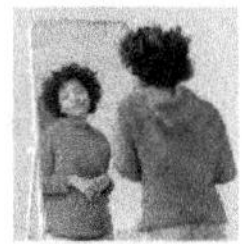

Take a moment to consider:

What stress management strategies have you tried in the past?

Which of these strategies resonate with you as potential tools for building resilience?

This week, choose two or three strategies from the list above and commit to incorporating them into your daily routine. Notice how they affect your stress levels and overall emotional well-being.

Building emotional resilience is an ongoing journey that requires intention and practice. By implementing these strategies, you can enhance your ability to manage stress effectively and cultivate a greater sense of well-being in your life.

Week 2: Physical & Mental Improvement

I invite you to explore my accompanying KDP planner, <u>The 40-Day Solitude Planner </u> (Available at amazon KDP)),_designed to enhance your journey through this experience. This planner not only helps you organize your thoughts and daily reflections but also serves as a creative space where you can track your progress and insights throughout the 40 days.

Day 8: Reflect on how your mind feels at the start of this week. Are there any mental stresses you'd like to let go of?

Day 9: Consider your sources of mental stimulation. What activities could help you expand your thinking?

Day 10: Reflect on your ability to focus. Are there distractions you can reduce?

Day 11: Identify a mental habit you'd like to improve. How can you start making this change?

Day 12: Think about how physical activity impacts your mood. Are there new activities you'd like to try?

Day 13: Reflect on any moments this week when you felt especially mentally clear. What contributed to that feeling?

Day 14: Look back on the week. How has combining physical and mental improvements affected you?

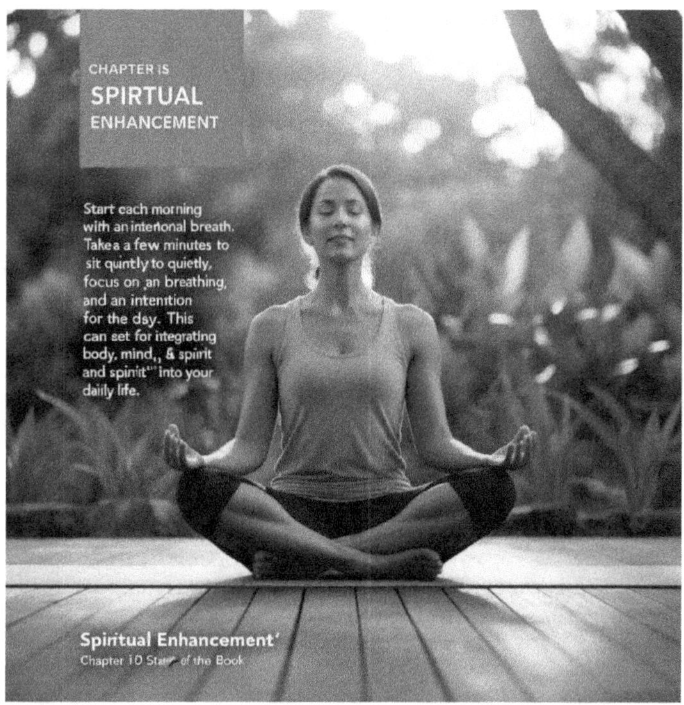

Chapter 4: Spiritual Enhancement

Have you ever felt a longing for something deeper in your life? A sense that your spirit craves renewal, much like the earth thirsts for rain after a long drought? In this chapter, we will explore the profound journey of spiritual renewal through various practices, connections with nature, and the act of serving others. Let's embark on this transformative path together.

Exploring Spiritual Practices

Have you ever felt a longing for something deeper in your life? A sense that your spirit craves renewal, much like the earth thirsts for rain after a long drought? In this chapter, we will explore the profound journey of spiritual renewal through various practices, connections with nature, and the act of serving others. Let's embark on this transformative path together.

The Power of Prayer and Meditation

Prayer: A Bridge to the Divine

Prayer is a timeless practice that transcends cultures and religions, serving as a bridge between our hearts and the spiritual realm. It provides a means to express our innermost thoughts, desires, and gratitude. Whether structured or spontaneous, prayer can take many forms:

Structured Prayer: Many traditions have established prayers that are recited during specific times or occasions. These prayers often contain profound wisdom and connect us to the beliefs and values of our heritage. For example, the Lord's Prayer in Christianity or the Shema in Judaism encapsulates core spiritual principles.

Spontaneous Prayer: This form of prayer is more personal and can occur at any moment. It allows for open-hearted communication with the divine, where you can share your thoughts, fears, and hopes without any constraints. This type of prayer can be particularly powerful during times of struggle or uncertainty.

Cultural Elements: To enrich your prayer practice, consider incorporating symbols or rituals from different traditions. For instance:

Candles: Lighting a candle while praying can symbolize illumination and hope.

Incense: Burning incense can create a sacred atmosphere, helping to focus your mind and spirit.

Nature Elements: Using natural elements like stones or flowers can ground your prayers in the physical world, reminding you of the interconnectedness of all life.

Meditation: Cultivating Inner Peace

Meditation is another powerful tool for spiritual renewal. It allows us to quiet our minds and focus on the present moment, creating space for deeper self-awareness and connection to our spiritual selves. Here are some key aspects of meditation:

Mindfulness Meditation: This practice involves paying attention to your breath and observing your thoughts without judgment. By anchoring yourself in the present moment, you cultivate awareness and acceptance.

Guided Meditation: Utilizing recordings or apps can help ease you into meditation. These guided sessions often include visualizations or affirmations that promote relaxation and spiritual insight.

Movement-Based Meditation: Practices like yoga or Tai Chi integrate physical movement with mindfulness, allowing you to connect your body and spirit through intentional motion.

Reflection Prompt

To deepen your understanding of how prayer and meditation impact your life, take some time for self-reflection:

Exercise: Spend five minutes each day this week in prayer or meditation. As you engage in these practices, pay attention to how they make you feel. What thoughts arise? What emotions surface? After each session, jot down any insights or revelations in a journal. Consider questions such as:

-How does my body feel during prayer or meditation?

-What thoughts distract me, and how do I respond to them?

-Do I notice any shifts in my mood or perspective after these moments of stillness?

Personal Story

I remember a time when I felt overwhelmed by life's demands—work pressures, family responsibilities, and an ever-growing to-do list seemed to consume my every waking moment. In search of peace amidst the chaos, I decided to embark on a daily meditation practice.

At first, it was challenging to quiet my mind. Thoughts raced through my head like a whirlwind—worries about deadlines, reminders of chores left undone, even random musings about what to have for dinner! However, I persisted. Each day, I carved out just five minutes in the morning to sit quietly with my breath.

Over time, I began to notice changes. The initial chaos gave way to moments of clarity; I found myself more grounded and present throughout my day. The simple act of focusing on my breath became a sanctuary where I could recharge my spirit. This practice transformed not only my outlook on life but also my ability to respond thoughtfully rather than react impulsively.

Conclusion

Incorporating prayer and meditation into your daily routine can serve as powerful catalysts for spiritual renewal. These practices allow you to reconnect with your inner self while fostering a deeper relationship with the divine. As you explore these tools throughout this chapter, remember that everyone's journey is unique—embrace what resonates with you and adapt these practices to fit your personal spiritual path. This expanded section provides more depth on exploring spiritual practices through prayer and meditation while maintaining an engaging tone.

Creating a personalized prayer practice that combines elements from different cultures can be a deeply enriching experience, allowing you to draw on the wisdom and beauty of various traditions. Here's how you can craft a unique and meaningful prayer practice:

Research and Explore Various Prayer Traditions

Start by exploring different cultural and religious practices to find elements that resonate with you. Here are some traditions to consider:

Native American Traditions: Often incorporate nature, music, and dance into prayer. Consider using natural elements like feathers or stones in your practice, or even incorporating drumming or singing as a form of expression.

Asian Practices: Look into Zen meditation from Japan or Qigong from China, which emphasize mindfulness and movement. You might integrate mindful breathing or gentle movements into your prayer routine.

Indigenous African Religions: These often involve communal chanting and dance, emphasizing connection with ancestors and the community. You could include rhythmic chanting or group prayers if you have a community to join.

Abrahamic Religions: Christianity, Judaism, and Islam offer structured prayers that can be adapted. For example, the Lord's Prayer or the Salah can serve as a framework while allowing for personal additions.

Incorporate Rituals and Symbols

Rituals and symbols can enhance your prayer practice by providing a tangible connection to your intentions:

Candles: Lighting a candle can symbolize illumination and intention. You might choose different colors based on what you wish to invoke (e.g., white for purity, green for healing).

Incense: Burning incense can create a sacred atmosphere. Different scents can evoke various feelings—lavender for calmness, sandalwood for grounding.

Nature Elements: Use items from nature such as flowers, stones, or water. For example, creating an altar with these elements can serve as a focal point during your prayers.

Create a Structure for Your Prayer Practice

While personalizing your practice, consider establishing a structure that incorporates various elements:

Set an Intention: Before beginning your prayer, take a moment to clarify what you seek—guidance, peace, gratitude, etc.

Combine Different Prayer Forms: Start with a structured prayer from one tradition (like the Lord's Prayer), then transition into spontaneous prayer where you express your personal thoughts and feelings.

Incorporate Meditation: After your prayer, spend time in silence or meditation to reflect on what you've expressed and to listen for any insights.

Engage in Community Practices

If possible, participate in community gatherings that reflect diverse spiritual practices:

Join Interfaith Groups: Look for local interfaith organizations that host prayer circles or meditation sessions. This exposure can introduce you to new practices and perspectives.

Volunteer for Community Service: Engage in service opportunities that align with various cultural traditions. This not only enriches your spiritual practice but also connects you with others who share similar values.

Reflect and Adapt

As you develop your personalized prayer practice, take time to reflect on its impact:

Journaling: Keep a journal of your experiences. Write about what resonates with you, what feels meaningful, and any insights gained during your prayers.

Be Open to Change: Your spiritual needs may evolve over time. Don't hesitate to adapt your practice by adding new elements or removing those that no longer serve you.

Conclusion

By combining elements from different cultures into your personalized prayer practice, you create a rich tapestry of spiritual expression that reflects your unique journey. Embrace the diversity of traditions while remaining respectful of their origins. This approach not only deepens your connection to the divine but also fosters appreciation for the myriad ways people seek spiritual fulfillment around the world.

Call to Action

Take some time this week to research at least two different cultural prayer practices that interest you. Experiment with incorporating one element from each into your own prayer routine. Reflect on how these additions impact your spiritual experience! This response provides a detailed guide on how to create a personalized prayer practice using elements from different cultures while incorporating actionable steps and reflection prompts.

In multicultural societies, fusion prayer practices often emerge, blending elements from different traditions to create new forms of spiritual expression. Here are some notable examples of how diverse cultural influences can come together in prayer:

Interfaith Prayer Circles

In many urban areas, interfaith prayer circles bring together individuals from different religious backgrounds to pray and meditate collectively. These gatherings often incorporate elements from each participant's tradition, such as:

-Christian prayers alongside Buddhist meditation techniques.

-Jewish blessings followed by Hindu chants or mantras.

-Muslim supplications integrated with Native American rituals, such as drumming or storytelling.

These circles foster a sense of community and mutual respect, allowing participants to share their spiritual practices while learning from one another.

Cultural Syncretism in Religious Practices

Religious syncretism occurs when elements from different religious traditions are combined to form new beliefs or practices. Some examples include:

Vodou in Haiti: This religion blends African spiritual practices with Catholicism, incorporating prayers to both African deities and Catholic saints. Rituals may involve offerings and prayers that reflect this dual heritage.

Candomblé in Brazil: Emerging during the transatlantic slave trade, Candomblé combines African beliefs with Christian elements. Practitioners honor orixás (spirits) associated with Catholic saints, creating a rich tapestry of prayer and ritual.

Sikhism: Originating in the Indian subcontinent, Sikhism combines elements of Hinduism and Islam, emphasizing monotheism and equality. The practice of prayer within Sikhism often includes reciting hymns from the Guru Granth Sahib, which reflects influences from both traditions.

Fusion Weddings

Multicultural weddings often feature fusion prayer practices that honor the couple's diverse backgrounds. For example:

-A couple might incorporate Jewish blessings and Hindu rituals into their wedding ceremony. This could include lighting a unity candle (a Christian tradition) alongside a sacred fire ceremony (a Hindu practice), symbolizing the merging of their lives and cultures.

-In a wedding that blends African American and Latino traditions, the ceremony might include communal prayers in both English and Spanish, alongside traditional songs that reflect both heritages.

Mindfulness and Meditation Practices

In modern Western societies, there is a growing trend towards integrating mindfulness and meditation into spiritual practices, reflecting a synthesis of Eastern practices with secular spirituality:

Many individuals now incorporate mindfulness meditation into their prayer routines, focusing on breath awareness while also reciting affirmations or prayers from various traditions.

Yoga classes often conclude with a moment of silent reflection or prayer that draws on different cultural influences, allowing practitioners to connect spiritually while engaging in physical movement.

Conclusion

Fusion prayer practices in multicultural societies exemplify the adaptability and richness of spiritual expression. By blending elements from various traditions, individuals can create personalized practices that resonate with their unique identities while fostering community and understanding among diverse groups. These practices not only enhance personal spirituality but also promote inclusivity and respect for different cultural backgrounds. This overview highlights examples of fusion prayer practices in multicultural contexts while emphasizing the importance of diversity in spiritual expression.

Fostering Connection with Nature

Have you ever felt a sense of peace wash over you while walking through a forest or sitting by a lake? Nature has an incredible ability to ground us, offering solace and inspiration. Fostering a connection with the natural world can enhance your spiritual renewal and promote mindfulness.

The Importance of Connecting with Nature

Spending time in nature has profound benefits for our mental, emotional, and spiritual well-being:

Reduces Stress: Nature has a calming effect, helping to lower cortisol levels and reduce anxiety.

Enhances Mood: Exposure to natural environments can boost your mood and increase feelings of happiness.

Promotes Mindfulness: Being in nature encourages us to be present, allowing us to engage our senses and appreciate the beauty around us.

Activities That Promote Mindfulness in Natural Settings

1. Nature Walks

Walking in nature is one of the simplest ways to connect with the environment. Here's how to make it mindful:

Choose a peaceful location, such as a park or hiking trail.

As you walk, pay attention to the sights, sounds, and smells around you. Notice the colors of the leaves, the rustling of branches, and the scent of fresh earth.

Take deep breaths and allow yourself to feel grounded in the moment.

2. Mindful Gardening

Gardening is a wonderful way to connect with nature while nurturing plants. To practice mindfulness while gardening:

Focus on the sensations of digging in the soil, feeling the texture of leaves, and observing how plants grow.

Use this time to reflect on your thoughts or simply enjoy the rhythm of your movements.

3. Meditation Outdoors

Find a quiet spot in nature where you can meditate. Here's a simple approach:

- ✓ Sit comfortably on the ground or a bench.

- ✓ Close your eyes and take several deep breaths.

- ✓ Focus on the sounds of nature—birds chirping, wind rustling through trees—and let these sounds anchor you in the present moment.

4. Nature Journaling

Keep a journal dedicated to your experiences in nature. This activity encourages reflection and creativity:

Write about your observations during walks or outdoor meditations.

Sketch or paint scenes from nature that inspire you.

I vividly recall a weekend spent camping in the mountains. Initially overwhelmed by my busy thoughts, I decided to take a solitary hike at sunrise. As I walked along the trail, I

became captivated by the golden light filtering through the trees. Each step felt lighter as I breathed in the crisp morning air. That experience reminded me that nature has an extraordinary way of bringing clarity and peace when we take time to truly connect with it.

Take a moment to reflect on your own relationship with nature:

How often do you spend time outdoors?

What activities can you incorporate into your routine to foster a deeper connection with nature?

Commit to spending at least 30 minutes outdoors each day. Choose one mindful activity from this section and immerse yourself fully in the experience. Notice how it affects your mood and sense of connection.

Fostering a connection with nature is essential for spiritual renewal. By engaging in mindful activities outdoors, you can enhance your well-being while cultivating a deeper appreciation for the world around you.

Here are some unique activities that promote mindfulness in nature, drawn from the search results:

Unique Mindfulness Activities in Nature

Forest Bathing (Shinrin-Yoku):

Immerse yourself in a forest environment, taking slow, deliberate steps while engaging your senses. Breathe deeply, listen to the sounds of rustling leaves and birds, and feel the textures of tree bark. This practice reduces stress and enhances your connection to nature.

Nature Journaling:

Bring a journal or sketchbook to a quiet spot in nature. Observe your surroundings closely and document your thoughts, sketches, or reflections. This activity encourages mindfulness and creativity while fostering a deeper appreciation for the natural world.

Mindful Gardening:

Engage in gardening by planting seeds or watering flowers. Focus on the sensations of the soil—the texture, temperature, and moisture—as well as the sounds and sights around you. This hands-on activity connects you with nature and promotes relaxation.

Sensory Exploration:

Find a tree or plant and explore its textures with your hands. Feel the roughness of bark or the softness of leaves. Engage all your senses by walking barefoot on grass or sand, splashing in water, or running blades of grass across your skin.

Nature Art:

Collect natural objects such as leaves, stones, and flowers to create art. Arrange them into shapes or patterns on the ground. This creative expression allows you to engage with nature while promoting mindfulness.

Mindful Walking:

Take a walk outdoors while focusing on each step you take. Pay attention to how your feet feel against different surfaces—grass, dirt, or gravel—and notice the rhythm of your breath as you walk.

Mindful Breathing Outdoors:

Find a comfortable spot outside and practice mindful breathing. Close your eyes and focus on inhaling the fresh air while listening to the sounds around you—birds chirping, leaves rustling—allowing yourself to be fully present in the moment.

Cloud Watching:

Lie down on the grass and watch the clouds roll by. Allow your mind to wander as you observe their shapes and movements, practicing mindfulness by being aware of your thoughts without judgment.

Wildlife Observation:

Spend time quietly observing wildlife in their natural habitat. Use binoculars if available, but simply watching animals can enhance your awareness of their behaviors and interactions.

Five Senses Scavenger Hunt:

Create a scavenger hunt that engages all five senses. Look for specific colors or shapes, listen for different sounds, smell flowers or plants, touch various textures, and even taste edible plants if safe to do so.

Rock Balancing:

Find smooth stones and challenge yourself to balance them on top of each other. This activity requires focus and patience, allowing you to practice mindfulness as you concentrate on achieving balance.

Nature Photography:

Use a camera or smartphone to capture images of nature that inspire you. Focus on details like textures, colors, and patterns to enhance your connection with your surroundings.

Mindful Picnicking:

Have a picnic where you practice mindful eating. Focus on the flavors and textures of your food while appreciating the sights and sounds around you.

Water Play:

If near a body of water, engage in water play by splashing or simply feeling the water against your skin. Enhance this experience with scented herbs or flowers for added sensory engagement.

Nature Meditation:

Find a tranquil spot outdoors where you can sit comfortably and meditate, focusing on the sounds of nature—like wind through trees or flowing water—to quiet your mind.

These activities not only promote mindfulness but also deepen your connection with nature, enhancing both mental clarity and emotional well-being.

Serving Others as a Path to Fulfillment

Have you ever experienced the joy of helping someone in need? That warm feeling in your heart, the sense of purpose—it's no coincidence. Serving others not only benefits those around us but also enhances our own spiritual growth. In this section, we'll explore the importance of community service and how it can lead to a more fulfilling life.

The Importance of Community Service

Engaging in community service provides numerous benefits that contribute to spiritual renewal:

1. Connection to Others

Serving others fosters a sense of belonging and connection. When you engage in acts of kindness, you build relationships with those in your community, creating a support network that enriches your life.

2. Increased Empathy and Compassion

Volunteering exposes you to diverse perspectives and experiences. This exposure cultivates empathy and compassion, allowing you to understand the struggles of others and appreciate your own circumstances more fully.

3. Sense of Purpose

Helping others gives your life meaning and direction. When you contribute to something larger than yourself, you cultivate a sense of purpose that can guide your decisions and actions.

4. Personal Growth

Community service challenges you to step outside your comfort zone. Whether it's learning new skills or confronting difficult situations, these experiences foster personal growth and resilience.

5. Enhanced Well-Being

Research shows that helping others can lead to improved mental health. Acts of kindness release endorphins, leading to what is often referred to as the "helper's high." This boost in mood can enhance your overall well-being.

Ways to Serve Others

1. Volunteer at Local Organizations

Find local charities or non-profits that resonate with your values. Whether it's serving meals at a soup kitchen, tutoring children, or participating in environmental clean-ups, there are countless opportunities to make a difference.

2. Participate in Community Events

Join community events such as fundraisers, awareness campaigns, or neighborhood clean-up days. These activities not only benefit the community but also allow you to meet like-minded individuals.

3. Offer Your Skills

Consider how your unique skills can benefit others. If you're good at graphic design, offer to create promotional materials for a local charity. If you have teaching experience, consider offering free workshops or classes.

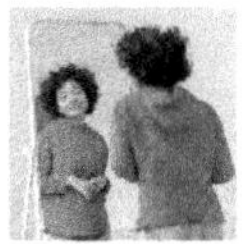

I remember my first experience volunteering at a local shelter. Initially hesitant, I was unsure how I could make an impact. However, as I served meals and interacted with guests, I realized that my presence alone brought smiles and gratitude. That experience opened my eyes to the power of service; it wasn't just about giving—it was about connecting and sharing humanity.

Take a moment to think about:

What causes resonate with you?

How have past experiences shaped your desire to serve others?

Commit to one act of service—big or small. Whether it's volunteering for a few hours or simply helping a neighbour, notice how it makes you feel and the connections you create.

Serving others is a powerful path toward spiritual renewal and fulfillment. By engaging in community service, you not only enrich the lives of those around you but also discover deeper meaning and purpose in your own life.

Week 3: Physical, Mental & Spiritual Improvement

Day 15: Reflect on what spirituality means to you. How can you integrate it into your solitude practice?

Day 16: Consider the connection between your body, mind, and spirit. How do they influence each other?

Day 17: Reflect on a moment that felt meaningful today. How can you create more of these moments?

Day 18: Think about gratitude. What are you grateful for in your life right now?

Day 19: Identify one spiritual value that resonates with you. How can you embody it in your daily life?

Day 20: Reflect on any feelings of inner peace you experienced this week. What led to those moments?

Day 21: Review the week. How has adding spiritual reflection impacted your journey?

Encouragement: You're embracing a holistic approach that's already enhancing your connection to yourself. Spiritual growth isn't always immediate, but each moment of quiet adds up. Be patient and let each small act of intention bring you peace.

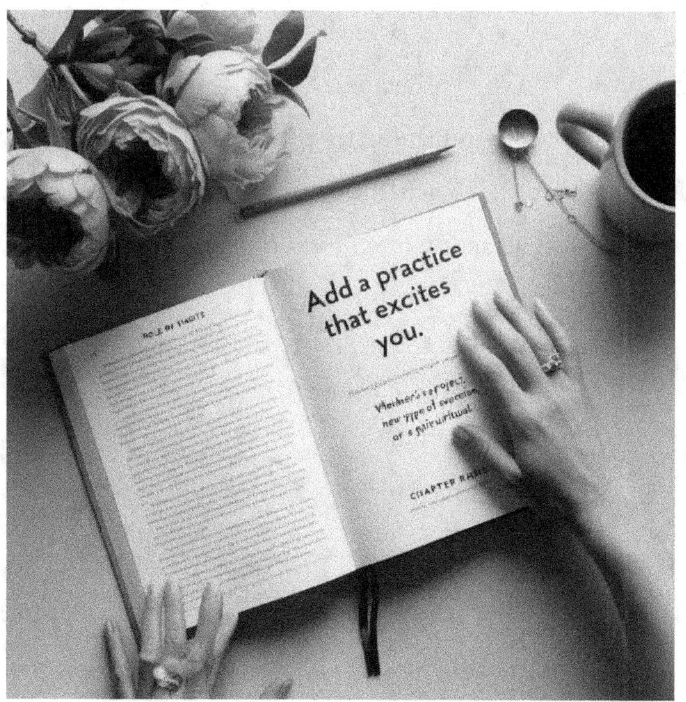

Chapter 5: Understanding the Role of Habits

The Science of Habit Formation

Have you ever wondered why you reach for your phone the moment you wake up, or why you automatically grab a snack when you sit down to watch TV? These behaviors are not random; they are habits formed through a fascinating process in our brains. Understanding how habits are formed and changed can empower you to create positive changes in your life.

How Habits Are Formed

The Three-Step Loop of Habit Formation

At the core of habit formation is a neurological pattern known as the habit loop, which consists of three key components:

Cue: This is the trigger that initiates the habit. It can be anything from a specific time of day, an emotional state, or an environmental cue. For example, seeing your running shoes might remind you to go for a jog.

Routine: This is the behavior itself—the action you take in response to the cue. It can be physical, mental, or emotional. For instance, if your cue is feeling stressed, your routine might be to reach for a snack.

Reward: The reward is what reinforces the habit and helps your brain determine whether this loop is worth remembering for the future. Rewards can be immediate (like the taste of chocolate) or delayed (like feeling accomplished after completing a workout).

As this loop repeats over time, it becomes more automatic, allowing your brain to conserve energy by not having to think about each action consciously.

Why Habits Emerge

Habits emerge because our brains are wired to seek efficiency. By automating certain behaviors, we free up mental resources for other tasks. This instinct to save effort is beneficial; it allows us to navigate daily life without constantly thinking about every action we take.

Changing Habits: The Golden Rule of Habit Change

To change a habit, you don't need to eradicate it; instead, you can replace it by keeping the same cue and reward but altering the routine. For example:

Current Habit: Snacking while watching TV (cue: sitting down to watch TV; routine: eating snacks; reward: enjoyment).

New Habit: Replacing snacks with herbal tea (same cue and reward but different routine).

Belief and Support

For a habit change to stick, it's crucial to believe that change is possible. Often, this belief is strengthened through support from others—whether friends, family, or community groups.

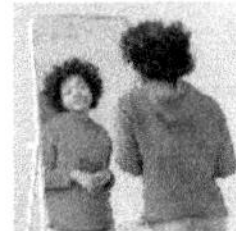

When I decided to improve my health by exercising regularly, I struggled to maintain motivation. I identified my cue as coming home from work and feeling tired. Instead of collapsing on the couch, I set up my workout clothes next to my front door as a visual cue. The new routine became changing into my workout gear immediately upon entering my home. The reward was not just the endorphins from exercising but also the satisfaction of sticking to my commitment. Over time, this new routine became automatic!

Take a moment to consider:

What habits do you have that serve you well?

Which habits would you like to change or replace?

Identify one habit you want to change. Use the habit loop framework (cue, routine, reward) to analyze it and create a plan for replacing it with a healthier behavior.

Understanding the science of habit formation empowers you to take control of your behaviors. By recognizing cues and rewards and applying strategies for change, you can cultivate positive habits that enhance your life.

Identifying Limiting Habits

Have you ever found yourself stuck in a cycle of behaviors that leave you feeling drained and unfulfilled? Recognizing limiting habits is the first step toward reclaiming your balance and enhancing your well-being. In this section, we'll explore exercises to help you identify habits that contribute to imbalance in your life.

Understanding Limiting Habits

Limiting habits are behaviors that hinder your growth, drain your energy, or create negative patterns in your life. They may manifest as procrastination, excessive screen time, unhealthy eating, or negative self-talk. Identifying these habits is crucial for making positive changes.

Exercises for Recognizing Limiting Habits

1. Daily Habit Journal

Keep a journal for one week where you track your daily habits. Note the following:

-What habits do you engage in regularly?

-How do these habits make you feel physically and emotionally?

-Are there any patterns or triggers associated with these habits?

At the end of the week, review your entries to identify any limiting habits that stand out.

2. The 5-Whys Technique

Choose one habit you suspect may be limiting. Ask yourself "Why?" five times to dig deeper into the root cause. For example:

Habit: I often snack mindlessly while watching TV.

Why? Because I feel bored. Why?

This exercise helps uncover underlying issues that contribute to limiting habits.

3. Mindfulness Reflection

Set aside a few moments each day for mindfulness reflection:

-Find a quiet space and take a few deep breaths.

-Reflect on your day and identify moments when you engaged in limiting habits.

-Consider how these habits affected your mood, energy levels, and overall well-being.

4. Visualizing Your Best Self

Create a vision board or write a description of your ideal self—how you want to feel, act, and live. Compare this vision to your current habits:

-What limiting habits are holding you back from becoming that person?

-What changes can you make to align more closely with your ideal self?

When I began my journey of self-improvement, I realized that my habit of scrolling through social media late at night was affecting my sleep and overall mood. To address this, I started journaling about my daily activities and feelings. This practice helped me see how much time I wasted online instead of pursuing hobbies or spending quality time with loved ones. Recognizing this limiting habit was eye-opening and motivated me to set boundaries around my screen time.

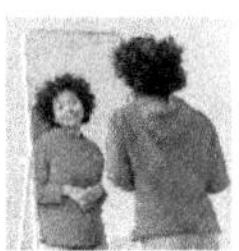

Take a moment to consider:

What are three habits that may be limiting your potential?

How do these habits impact your daily life?

This week, choose one exercise from above to help identify a limiting habit in your life. Write down what you discover and reflect on actionable steps you can take to change it.

Identifying limiting habits is essential for achieving balance and enhancing your well-being. By engaging in these exercises, you can gain clarity on the behaviors that hold you back and begin taking steps toward positive change.

Week 4: Consistency with Physical, Mental & Spiritual Habits

Day 22: Reflect on your progress so far. What habits have started to feel natural?

Day 23: Consider a challenge you've encountered. What mindset shift might help you overcome it?

Day 24: Reflect on how your solitude practices have affected your physical health. What feels different?

Day 25: Think about your mental resilience. What has helped strengthen your mind during this journey?

Day 26: Reflect on your spiritual growth. How has solitude helped you deepen your understanding?

Day 27: Identify one thing you'd like to continue improving. What small step can you take today?

Day 28: Look back over the week. How have consistency and discipline shaped your experience?

Encouragement: Consistency is key, and you're doing an incredible job building habits that truly serve you. Embrace any challenges as part of the journey—they're shaping your commitment and making these practices feel more natural and fulfilling.

Week 5: Deepening & Expanding Your Routine

Day 29: Reflect on your daily solitude routine. What elements feel most meaningful to you?

Day 30: Think about the role of self-compassion. How can you treat yourself with more kindness in this process?

Day 31: Reflect on a habit that feels challenging. What can you do to make it more enjoyable?

Day 32: Identify a new practice you want to explore. How might it contribute to your physical, mental, or spiritual health?

Day 33: Reflect on your current motivations. What drives you to continue with this journey?

Day 34: Consider how you might share your growth with others. How can your experience inspire those around you?

Day 35: Review the week. What progress have you made in deepening your connection with solitude?

You've come so far! By exploring new ways to grow, you're not just maintaining these practices—you're making them a rewarding part of your life. Every bit of dedication and curiosity you bring strengthens your renewal journey.

Week 6: Integrating Habits for Lifelong Renewal

Day 36: Reflect on the journey you've taken over these six weeks. What stands out as most transformative?

Day 37: Consider how these new habits have shaped your perspective. What feels different?

Day 38: Reflect on how you can maintain this renewal in everyday life. What practices feel essential to carry forward?

Day 39: Think about the challenges you may face after this program. How will you stay committed to your renewal?

Day 40: Reflect on the power of solitude. How has this experience prepared you to embrace solitude as a lifelong ally?

This journey has been transformative, and you've built something truly meaningful. Trust that these practices will continue to guide and empower you, keeping you grounded and renewed for the long run. You're ready to carry this growth forward!

Habit-Building Toolkit: Takeaway for Lasting Transformation

Congratulations on completing your 40-day journey! This toolkit is designed to help you carry forward the habits you've cultivated, ensuring they remain a core part of your daily life.

1. Set Clear Intentions and Goals

Define Your 'Why': Understanding why a habit is important gives it purpose and keeps you motivated, even on difficult days. Reflect on what each habit brings to your life, whether it's physical strength, mental clarity, or spiritual peace.

SMART Goals: Revisit the SMART framework—specific, measurable, achievable, relevant, and time-bound. Setting well-defined goals helps turn abstract intentions into actionable steps.

2. Build a Habit-Stacking Routine

Link New Habits to Existing Routines: Make new habits easier to remember by pairing them with established routines. For example, if you already have a morning coffee ritual, add 5 minutes of deep breathing right afterward.

Use 'Cue-Action-Reward' Loops: Habits are more likely to stick when they have a clear trigger, a consistent action, and a satisfying reward. Identify a cue for each habit, such as a time of day, and reward yourself with something simple—a moment of relaxation or a Favorite activity.

3. Track Your Progress

Daily Journal or Log: Keeping a journal or log of your habits allows you to visually track your progress and see how far you've come. Note how each habit impacts your physical, mental, and spiritual well-being.

Habit Tracking Tools: Use a habit-tracking app or a physical calendar to monitor consistency. Seeing your progress builds motivation, and noticing when you miss a day allows you to quickly get back on track.

4. Stay Accountable and Connected

Accountability Partner: Find a friend or loved one who can check in with you. Sharing your progress and setbacks can help keep you committed.

Join a Supportive Community: Consider joining our Telegram channel; <u>Alone for 40 Days,</u> dedicated to the "Alone for 40 Days" journey. Engage with others who are also focused on growth, share insights, and encourage each other on the path.

5. Practice Self-Compassion

Allow for Imperfection: Habit-building is a gradual process, and there may be days when you slip. Rather than feeling discouraged, view setbacks as part of the journey and focus on recommitting to your goals.

Celebrate Small Wins: Recognize and celebrate every small step forward. This creates a positive association with the habit and reinforces your commitment.

6. Adapt and Evolve

Review and Reflect Monthly: Regularly evaluate your habits to ensure they still serve your needs and align with your goals. If something no longer feels beneficial, consider tweaking it or trying a new approach.

Embrace New Challenges: Keep your routine fresh by introducing occasional changes. Trying a new activity, like a creative project or a different mindfulness technique, can keep the journey engaging and support continuous growth.

This Habit-Building Toolkit serves as a foundation to help you sustain the growth you've achieved over the past 40 days. Remember, the journey doesn't end here; it's just the beginning of a life enriched by solitude, mindfulness, and purposeful habits. May these tools guide and inspire you to keep building a life that nurtures your physical, mental, and spiritual well-being.

Conclusion: Reflecting on Foundations

As we reach the end of Part 1, it's essential to pause and reflect on the foundational insights we've explored together. Each chapter has contributed to a holistic understanding of personal renewal, emphasizing the interconnectedness of physical, mental, and spiritual well-being.

Key Insights from the Book

1. Physical Renewal

We began our journey by recognizing the significance of rest and recovery. Prioritizing sleep, nutrition, and exercise is not merely about physical health; it's about creating a solid foundation for all other aspects of our lives. When our bodies are well-cared for, we have the energy and vitality to pursue our goals and navigate challenges.

2. Mental Improvement

Next, we delved into cultivating mindfulness and awareness. By practicing mindfulness techniques, we enhance our ability to focus, reduce stress, and foster emotional resilience. This mental clarity allows us to engage more fully with our experiences and make intentional choices that align with our values.

3. Spiritual Enhancement

We explored the importance of connecting with nature and fostering a sense of spirituality. Nature serves as a powerful reminder of our place in the world and can provide solace during turbulent times. By nurturing this connection, we cultivate a deeper sense of purpose and fulfillment in our lives.

4. Understanding the Role of Habits

Finally, we examined the science of habit formation. Understanding how habits are formed empowers us to create positive changes in our lives. By setting realistic goals and breaking them down into manageable steps, we can build sustainable practices that support our journey of renewal.

Moving Forward

As you reflect on these insights, take a moment to consider how they apply to your own life:

What practices resonate most with you?

How can you prioritize physical, mental, and spiritual renewal in your daily routine?

What small steps can you take to integrate these insights into your life moving forward?

Embrace this opportunity for reflection as a catalyst for growth. The foundations you've built in Part 1 are essential as you prepare to embark on the next phase of your journey—where application and integration will lead to meaningful transformation.

CALL TO ACTION   Take a few moments to journal your thoughts on these questions or discuss them with a friend or mentor.

The 40-Day Approach – A Transformational Guide

Why 40 Days?

The concept of dedicating 40 days to a transformative journey is rooted in both historical and spiritual significance. This time frame has been recognized across various cultures and religions as a period of profound change, reflection, and renewal.

Historical and Spiritual Significance of 40 Days

Biblical References:

-In the Bible, the number 40 appears frequently as a period of testing, trial, and preparation. For example: Moses

-These examples illustrate that 40 days often signifies a time of significant transformation, spiritual awakening, and preparation for what lies ahead.

Cultural Significance:

Many cultures have recognized the power of a defined period for change. For instance, some indigenous traditions use similar time frames for vision quests or rites of passage, emphasizing introspection and personal growth.

Personal Reflection:

Dedicating 40 days allows individuals to step away from their daily routines and distractions. This intentional focus can lead to deeper insights and a more profound understanding of oneself.

The Psychology Behind Habit Formation and Commitment

The 21/90 Rule:

While many believe it takes 21 days to form a habit, research suggests that it typically takes longer—around 66 days on average—to establish a new behavior as automatic. The 40-day approach falls within this range, providing ample time for individuals to practice new habits consistently.

Commitment and Accountability:

Committing to a structured period like 40 days creates a sense of accountability. Knowing that you are dedicating this time to self-improvement can enhance motivation and commitment.

Setting clear goals for this period encourages individuals to track their progress and reflect on their journey regularly.

Reinforcement of Positive Behaviors:

Engaging in new practices daily over the course of 40 days reinforces positive behaviors. The repetition helps solidify these habits in your routine, making it easier to maintain them long after the initial commitment ends.

How 40 Days Allows for Comprehensive Renewal

Holistic Transformation:

The 40-day approach allows for comprehensive renewal by addressing multiple aspects of life—physical, mental, emotional, and spiritual. This holistic focus ensures that changes are not superficial but rather deeply integrated into one's lifestyle.

Time for Reflection:

With each passing day, individuals have the opportunity to reflect on their experiences, challenges, and successes. This reflection fosters deeper self-awareness and understanding, paving the way for meaningful growth.

Building Resilience:

Committing to a transformative journey over 40 days can help build resilience. As individuals face obstacles and learn to navigate them, they develop coping strategies that enhance their ability to handle future challenges.

Creating Lasting Change:

By dedicating this time to personal renewal, individuals are more likely to create lasting change in their lives. The insights gained during this period can serve as a foundation for ongoing growth and self-discovery.

Embracing the 40-day approach offers a unique opportunity for transformation. By understanding its historical significance, leveraging psychological principles of habit formation, and committing to comprehensive renewal, you can embark on a powerful journey toward self-discovery and lasting change. Whether you seek physical health, mental clarity, or spiritual connection, dedicating these 40 days can set you on a path toward a more fulfilling life.

**The End, Journey continues go forth
with courage and determination**

Mind Map: Alone for 40 Days

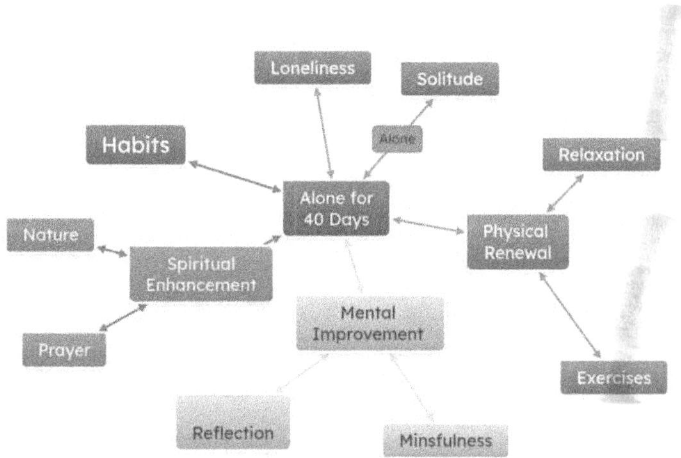